Your Keto Cooking Guide

*Delicious & Tasty Recipes for Your Keto Diet
Daily Meals to Burn Fat and Boost your
Metabolism*

Diana Ramos

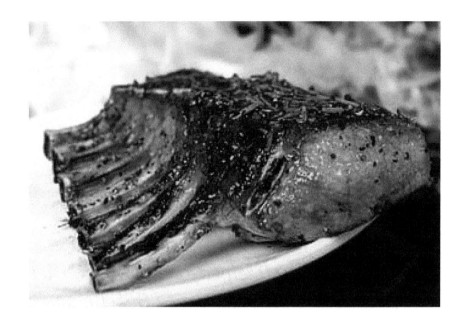

present accurate, up to date, and reliable, complete information. No warranties of any kind are declared or implied. Readers acknowledge that the author is not engaging in the rendering of legal, financial, medical or professional advice. The content within this book has been derived from various sources. Please consult a licensed professional before attempting any techniques outlined in this book.

By reading this document, the reader agrees that under no circumstances is the author responsible for any losses, direct or indirect, which are incurred as a result of the use of information contained within this document, including, but not limited to, — errors, omissions, or inaccuracies.

Table of Contents

Bacon-Wrapped Chicken Breasts Stuffed With Spinach

Macros: Fat 59% | Protein 39% | Carbs 2%

Prep time: 25 minutes | Cook time: 1 hour | Serves 4

Trust me, this easy bacon-wrapped chicken breasts stuffed with spinach will become your family favorite! The flavor of the cheeses will bring you and your families tons of flavor. And the choice of spinach for this recipe will also increase the nutritional value of the meal.

- 1 (10-ounce / 284-g) package frozen chopped spinach, thawed and drained
- ½ cup mayonnaise, keto-friendly
- ½ cup feta cheese, shredded
- 2 cloves garlic, chopped
- 4 skinless, boneless chicken breasts
- 4 slices bacon

Preheat the oven to 375ºF (190ºC).

Combine the spinach, mayo, feta cheese, and garlic in a bowl, then set aside.

Cut the chicken crosswise to butterfly the chicken breasts, (butterfly cutting technique: not to cut the chicken breast through, leave a 1-inch space uncut at the end of the chicken, and flipping open the halved chicken breast, it resembles a butterfly.

Unfold the chicken breasts like a book. Divide and arrange the spinach mixture over each breast, then wrap each breast with a slice of bacon and secure with a toothpick.

Arrange them in a baking dish, and cover a piece of aluminum foil. Place the dish in the preheated oven and bake for 1 hour or until the bacon is crispy and the juice of chicken breasts run clear.

Remove the baking dish from the oven and serve warm.

STORAGE: Store in an airtight container in the fridge for up to 4 days or in the freezer for up to 1 month.

REHEAT: Microwave, covered, until the desired temperature is reached or reheat in a frying pan or air fryer / instant pot, covered, on medium.

SERVE IT WITH: To make this a complete meal, serve them on a bed of greens or serve with a cherry tomato and zucchini salad.

PER SERVING

calories: 626 | fat: 41.3g | total carbs: 3.7g | fiber: 1.4g | protein: 61.2g

Rotisserie-Style Roast Chicken

Macros: Fat 64% | Protein 35% | Carbs 1%

Prep time:10minutes | Cook time: 5 hours | Serves 8

With minimal preparation and about 5 hours' cooking time,you can get that restaurant-style rotisserie chicken at home as you ever wish. It is super simple to make. No special skills are required. It is delicious and the leftovers are just as good the next day!

- 1teaspoon onion powder
- 1 teaspoon white pepper
- 1 teaspoon dried thyme
- ½ teaspoon garlic powder
- ½ teaspoon cayenne pepper
- 1 teaspoons paprika
- 2teaspoons salt
- ½ teaspoon black pepper
- 1 (4-pound / 1.8-kg) whole chickens, giblets removed, rinsed and pat dry
- 1 onion, quartered

Combine the onion powder, white pepper, thyme, garlic powder, cayenne pepper, paprika, salt, and black pepper in a bowl.

Rub the whole chicken with the powder mixture on all sides. Arrange the onion quarters into the cavity of the chicken.

Wrap the chicken with two layers of plastic and refrigerate for at least 4 hours.

Preheat the oven to 250°F (120°C).

Arrange the chicken in a baking pan and bake in the preheated oven for 5 hours or until a meat thermometer inserted in the chicken center reads at least 180°F (82°C).

Remove the chicken from the oven. Allow to cool for 10 minutes and   slice to serve.

STORAGE: Store in an airtight container in the fridge for up to 4 days or in the freezer for up to 1 month.

REHEAT: Microwave, covered, until the desired temperature is reached or reheat in a frying pan or air fryer / instant pot, covered, on medium.

SERVE IT WITH: Easy lemon-ginger spinach is a perfect match for this dish, or you can have it with oven-roasted frozen broccoli cooked in the left juices. It will burst the flavors inside your mouth.

PER SERVING

calories: 484 | fat: 34.2g | total carbs: 2.2g | fiber: 0.6g | protein: 42.5g

Chicken Fajitas Bake

Macros: Fat 74% | Protein 21% | Carbs 5%

Prep time: 10 minutes | Cook time: 15 minutes | Serves 4 to 6

This keto chicken casserole is the perfect low-carb meal for the whole family. It has all of your favorite fajita flavors all in one skillet. It is super simple, with only 7 main ingredients, and can be made in about 20 minutes. This would be a great weeknight family-friendly keto recipe. It's an easy keto recipe for beginners, too!

- ⅓ cup mayonnaise, keto-friendly
- 1 yellow onion, chopped
- 1 red bell pepper, chopped
- 1 rotisserie chicken breast, shred into bite-sized pieces
- 2 tablespoons Tex-Mex seasoning
- 2 tablespoons olive oil
- 5⅓ ounces (150 g) lettuce
- 7 ounces (198 g) cream cheese
- Salt and freshly ground black pepper, to taste
- 7 ounces (198 g) shredded Cheddar cheese, divided

Preheat the oven to 400°F (205°C).

Add all the ingredients except for a third of the cheese to a lightly greased casserole dish. Stir to combine well.

Top the mixture with remaining cheese, then arrange the casserole dish in the preheated oven. Bake for 15 minutes or until lightly browned.

Remove the casserole dish from the oven and serve warm.

STORAGE: Store in an airtight container in the fridge for up to 4 days.

REHEAT: Microwave, covered, until the desired temperature is reached or reheat in a frying pan or air fryer / instant pot, covered, on medium.

SERVE IT WITH: To make this a complete meal, you can serve this casserole dish with leafy greens dressed in olive oil.

PER SERVING

calories: 526 | fat: 43.1g | total carbs: 7.0g | fiber: 1.5g | protein: 27.7g

Savoury And Sticky Baked Chicken Wings

Macros: Fat 37% | Protein 62% | Carbs 1%

Prep time: 5 minutes | Cook time: 45 minutes | Serves 4

These wings are great. There is a heat to them, but non-spice lovers enjoy them too because of the sweetness. They have a sweet, spicy, smoky flavor that will make you do a happy dance for sure! Made with a keto-friendly homemade marinade you can ensure no nasty preservatives or refined sugars in these bad boys!

- 2 pounds (907 g) chicken wings
- 1 teaspoon sea salt

SAUCE:

- ¾ cup coconut aminos
- ¼ teaspoon garlic powder
- ¼ teaspoon red pepper flakes
- ¼ teaspoon onion powder
- ¼ teaspoon ground ginger

Preheat oven to 450°F (235°C).

Arrange the chicken wings in a baking pan, skin side down. Make sure to keep a little distance between wings.

Sprinkle salt to season the wings, then bake in the preheated oven for 45 minutes or until crispy and cooked through.

Meanwhile, make the sauce: Warm a nonstick skillet over medium heat, add the coconut aminos, garlic powder, red pepper flakes, onion powder, and ginger powder. Bring them to a simmer.

Reduce the heat to low and keep simmering. Stir the mixture constantly to combine well until the sauce is lightly thickened.

Arrange the chicken wings on a large serving dish. Pour the sauce over to coat the chicken wings and serve warm.

STORAGE: Store in an airtight container in the fridge for up to 4 days.

REHEAT: Microwave, covered, until the desired temperature is reached or reheat in a frying pan or air fryer / instant pot, covered, on medium.

SERVE IT WITH: Serve them with roasted Brussels sprout and rich cod fish soup.

PER SERVING

calories: 450 | fat: 18.5g | total carbs: 9.4g | fiber: 0.1g | protein: 69.2g

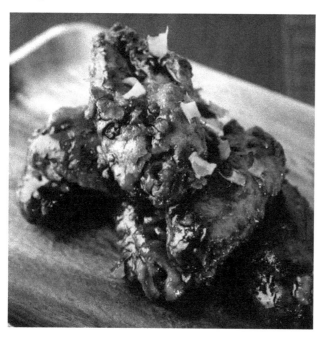

Low-Carb Chicken With Tricolore Roasted Veggies

Macros: Fat 71% | Protein 21% | Carbs 8%

Prep time: 15 minutes | Cook time: 30 minutes | Serves 8

It is a beautiful and most colorful dish. So easy-to-make with lots of good flavor, and you can choose to cook it with either a whole chicken or chicken breasts.

TRICOLORE ROASTED VEGGIES:

- 8 ounces (227 g) mushrooms
- 1 pound (454 g) Brussels sprouts
- 8 ounces (227 g) cherry tomatoes
- 1 teaspoon dried rosemary
- 1 teaspoon sea salt
- ½ teaspoon ground black pepper
- ½ cup olive oil

FRIED CHICKEN:

- 4 chicken breasts
- 1 ounce (28 g) butter, for frying
- Salt and freshly ground black pepper, to taste
- 4 ounces (113 g) herb butter, for serving

Preheat the oven to 400°F (205°C).

Arrange the mushrooms, Brussels sprouts, and cherry tomatoes in a baking pan.

Sprinkle with rosemary, salt, and ground black pepper. Pour the olive oil over. Stir to coat the veggies well.

Arrange the baking pan in the preheated oven and bake for about 20 minutes or until the Brussels sprouts are wilted and the veggies are soft.

In the meantime, melt the butter in a nonstick skillet over medium heat, then place the chicken breasts in the pan. Sprinkle with salt and pepper.

Fry the chicken in the skillet for 8 to 10 minutes or until there is no pink on the chicken and the juices run clear.

Remove the baked veggies from the oven and serve with the fried chicken.

STORAGE: Roasted vegetables can be stored in the refrigerator for 3 to 4 days. Store any leftover chicken in the fridge. This will store for up to three days.

REHEAT: Heat roasted vegetables again in a hot oven to keep them firm and crisp. A microwave will just turn them to mush. Spread the vegetables out on a baking sheet, drizzle them with olive oil, and bake at 450°F (235°C) for 4 or 5 minutes.

SERVE IT WITH: To make this a complete meal, you can serve it with with roasted Brussels sprout and rich sea white fish soup.

PER SERVING

calories: 390 | fat: 30.8g | total carbs: 10.4g | fiber: 3.1g | protein: 20.9g

Cheese Stuffed Chicken Breast With Guacamole

Macros: Fat 69% | Protein 23% | Carbs 8%

Prep time: 20 minutes | Cook time: 20 minutes | Serves 6

This is a super delicious recipe. The taste of cheese with the flavor of the spiced chicken is balanced, and the cheese can be changed to Parmesan cheese for additional salty flavor. This is a meal with low budget to maintain a healthy body.

CHEESE STUFFED CHICKEN:

- 1 green bell pepper or red bell pepper, chopped
- 1 garlic clove, granulated
- 2 tablespoons olive oil
- 1½ pounds (680 g) chicken breasts
- 3 ounces (85 g) cream cheese
- 4 ounces (113 g) Cheddar cheese, shredded
- 2 tablespoons pickled jalapeños, finely chopped
- ½ teaspoon ground cumin
- 1 ginger, minced
- Salt and freshly ground black pepper, to taste

SPECIAL EQUIPMENT:

4 toothpicks, soak in water for at least 30 minutes

FOR SERVING:

- 8 ounces (227 g) lettuce 1 cup sour cream

GUACAMOLE:

- 2 ripe avocados, peeled
- ½ lime, the juice
- 2garlic cloves, minced
- 1 diced tomato
- 3 tablespoons olive oil
- 5 tablespoons fresh cilantro, finely chopped
- Salt and freshly ground black pepper, to taste

Preheat the oven to 350°F (180°C).

Warm the olive oil in a nonstick skillet over medium heat. Add the garlic and bell pepper and sauté for about 3 minutes until the bell pepper is soft. Transfer to a bowl and allow to cool for 5 minutes.

Sprinkle the cheeses, jalapeños, cumin, and ginger in the bowl. Toss to combine well. Set aside.

Butterfly the chicken breasts by cutting them crosswise and leave a 1- inch space uncut at the end of the breasts.

Unfold the breasts on a clean working surface like a book, divide and spread the cheese mixture in the breasts. Close the 'book' and secure each chicken breast with a toothpick. Sprinkle with salt and pepper.

Arrange the stuffed chicken breasts in a lightly greased frying pan and fry for 8 minutes or until lightly browned. Place the fried chicken in a baking dish.

Pour the remaining cheese mixture over the chicken breasts and bake in the preheated oven for 20 minutes or until a meat thermometer inserted in the middle of the chicken reads at least 165°F (74°C).

Remove the toothpicks and serve with lettuce, guacamole, and sour cream.

GUACAMOLE:

Mash the guacamole with a fork in a large bowl. Top with lime juice and minced garlic.

Add tomato, olive oil and finely chopped cilantro. Season with salt and pepper, and blend well.

STORAGE: Chicken breast filled cheese with guacamole can be stored covered in the fridge for 2 up to 3 days, you can even freeze it in a freezer- safe container for up to 1 month.

REHEAT: Microwave, until it reaches the desired temperature.

SERVE IT WITH: To make it a complete meal, you can serve it with a mushroom and salmon salad and berry smoothie.

PER SERVING

calories: 599 | fat: 47.1g | total carbs: 13.5g | fiber: 5.9g | protein: 32.8g

Garlic Chicken Low-Carb

Macros: Fat 66% | Protein 31% | Carbs 3%

Prep time: 15 minutes | Cook time: 45 minutes | Serves 4

For those who look for simplicity, strong taste, and few calories, this recipe offers you great taste, distinct flavor, and simplicity of preparation.

- 2 ounces (57 g) butter
- 2 pounds (907 g) chicken drumsticks
- Salt and freshly ground black pepper, to taste ù
- 2 tablespoons olive oil
- 1 lemon, the juice
- 7 garlic cloves, sliced
- ½ cup fresh parsley, finely chopped

Start by preheating the oven to 450°F (235°C).

Grease the baking pan with butter and put the chicken drumsticks, season with salt and pepper generously.

Drizzle the olive oil and lemon juice over the chicken pieces. Sprinkle the garlic and parsley on top.

Bake the chicken for 30 to 40 minutes or until the garlic slices become golden and chicken pieces turn brown and roasted, the baking time may be longer if your drumsticks are on the large size. Lower the temperature considerably towards the end.

STORAGE: Low-carb garlic chicken can be stored in the fridge for 1 up to 4 days, it can even be kept in the freezer for 15 days.

REHEAT: Microwave, covered, until the desired temperature is reached or reheat in a frying pan or air fryer / instant pot, covered, on medium.

SERVE IT WITH: This wonderful recipe is served cold or hot, can be Serve with aioli and a hearty salad and toast with garlic. Some people favor it with a delectable cauliflower mash.

PER SERVING

calories: 542 | fat: 40.0g | total carbs: 4.0g | fiber: 1.0g | protein: 42.0g

Creamy Pork Loin and Mushrooms

Macros: Fat 53% | Protein 45% | Carbs 3%

Prep time: 10 minutes | Cook time: 20 minutes | Serves 4

This is a healthy dish. It is easy to cook and has a delicious taste. The group of mushrooms and pork is classic and the best. The pork is infused in the mushroom's fragrance; it gives you an amazing eating experience.

- 2 pounds (907 g) pork loin
- Salt and freshly ground black pepper, to taste
- 2 tablespoons butter
- 1 cup white mushrooms
- ¾ cup sour cream

In a bowl, add the pork. Add black pepper and salt to season.

In a nonstick skillet, add butter and heat over medium heat. Add the pork and sauté for 3 minutes.

Pour mushroom and sour cream over the pork. Put the lid on and cook for 15 minutes until the pork is cooked through.

Transfer to serving plates and serve while hot.

STORAGE: Store in an airtight container in the refrigerator for up to 4 days or in the freezer for up to 1 month.

REHEAT: Microwave, covered, until the desired temperature is reached or reheat in a frying pan or air fryer / instant pot, covered, on medium.

SERVE IT WITH: To make this a complete meal, serve with egg mayo salad.

PER SERVING

calories: 573 | fat: 33.6g | total carbs: 3.8g | fiber: 0.2g | protein: 60.6g

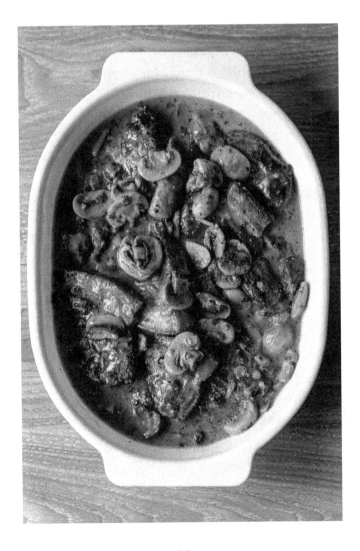

Pork Chops with Dijon Mustard

Macros: Fat 51% | Protein 48% | Carbs 1%

Prep time: 20 minutes | Cook time: 50 minutes | Serves 4

The delicacy is perfect for an easy weeknight dinner. The tender and crispy nature of the pork chops with mustard will enlighten your palate. It is tasty with an amazing rosemary flavor.

- 1 tablespoon olive oil
- 4 pork chops
- 2 tablespoons Dijon mustard
- 1 tablespoon fresh rosemary, coarsely chopped
- Salt and freshly ground black pepper, to taste
- 2 tablespoons butter

Preheat the oven to 350 °F (180 °C) and lightly grease a baking dish with olive oil.

In a bowl, add the pork chops. Add the mustard, rosemary, black pepper and salt. Toss to combine well. Wrap the bowl in plastic and refrigerate to marinate for at least 45 minutes.

Discard the marinade and transfer the pork chops to the baking dish and add the butter. Bake for 45 minutes until an instant-read thermometer inserted in the center of the pork registers at least 165°F (74°C).

Transfer to serving plates to serve while warm.

STORAGE: Store in an airtight container in the refrigerator for up to 4 days or in the freezer for up to 1 month.

REHEAT: Microwave, covered, until the desired temperature is reached or reheat in a frying pan or air fryer / instant pot, covered, on medium.

SERVE IT WITH: To make this a complete meal, serve with mushroom vegan kale salad.

PER SERVING

calories: 363 | fat: 21.0g | total carbs: 0.5g | fiber: 0.4g | protein: 40.5g

Beef and Buttered Brussels Sprouts

Macros: Fat 78% | Protein 18% | Carbs 4%

Prep time: 10 minutes | Cook time: 20 minutes | Serves 2

It is perfect for individuals who love simple meals as it has no complexities. The meal is easy to fix and with a tasty Brussels sprouts flavor.

- 1½ ounces (43 g) butter
- 5 ounces (142 g) ground beef
- 4½ ounces (128 g) Brussels sprouts
- Salt and freshly ground black pepper, to taste
- ¼ cup keto-friendly mayonnaise

In a large pan, add 3 tablespoons of butter and melt over medium heat.

Add the beef and cook until well browned for about 8 minutes.

Reduce the heat and add Brussels sprouts, black pepper, salt and the remaining butter. Cooks for 8 more minutes. Stir periodically.

Transfer the beef and Brussels sprouts to serving plates and top with keto-friendly mayonnaise before serving.

STORAGE: Store in an airtight container in the refrigerator for up to 4 days or in the freezer for up to 1 month.

REHEAT: Microwave, covered, until the desired temperature is reached or reheat in a frying pan or air fryer / instant pot, covered, on medium.

SERVE IT WITH: To make this a complete meal, serve with broccoli slaw.

PER SERVING

calories: 513 | fat: 44.8g | total carbs: 5.9g | fiber: 2.4g | protein: 22.3g

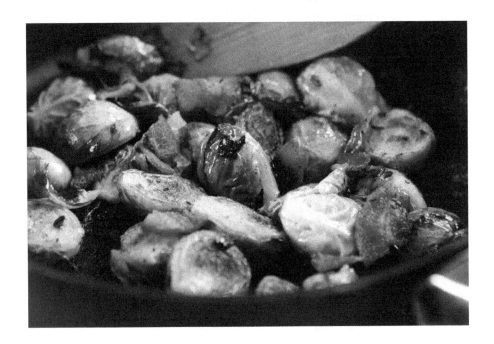

Garlicky Beef Steak

Macros: Fat 70% | Protein 29% | Carbs 1%

Prep time: 15 minutes | Cook time: 30 minutes | Serves 6

It is easy to cook and with an amazing creamy taste. The crispy nature just brings joy into eating beef steak. The ingredients of this recipe also give you a large space to try your idea out, you can make this recipe luscious.

- 2 pounds (907 g) sirloin beef top steaks
- 4 minced garlic cloves
- Salt and freshly ground black pepper, to taste
- ½ cup butter
- 1½ cups cream

On a clean board, add the beefsteak and rub with garlic, black pepper and salt.

Mix butter and cream in a bowl. Add the beef to the mixture. Wrap the bowl in plastic and refrigerate to marinate for at least 45 minutes.

Preheat the grill to medium-high heat.

Transfer the steaks to the grill and allow each side to grill for 10 minutes.

Transfer to serving plates and serve while hot.

STORAGE: Store in an airtight container in the refrigerator for up to 4 days or in the freezer for up to 1 month.

REHEAT: Microwave, covered, until the desired temperature is reached or reheat in a frying pan or air fryer/instant pot, covered, on medium.

SERVE IT WITH: To make this a complete meal, serve with mushroom avocado tuna salad.

PER SERVING

calories: 485 | fat: 38.2g | total carbs: 1.5g | fiber: 0g | protein: 32.6g

Seasoned Beef Roast

Macros: Fat 41% | Protein 57% | Carbs 2%

Prep time: 10 minutes | Cook time: 50 minutes | Serves 4

It is a perfect dish for a Sunday lunch. It's easy to cook and you can enjoy it with friends or family. You can store it for future use if you wish. The roast beef with broth will bring you a very nice taste.

- 2 pounds (907 g) beef roast
- 1 cup onion soup
- 1 cup beef broth
- Salt and freshly ground black pepper, to taste

Add beef roast in a pressure cooker. Add onion soup, beef broth, black pepper and salt. Cover the lid of the pressure cooker and cook for 50 minutes at high pressure.

Naturally release the pressure. Transfer to a serving plate to cool before serving.

STORAGE: Store in an airtight container in the refrigerator for up to 4 days.

REHEAT: Microwave, covered, until the desired temperature is reached or reheat in a frying pan or air fryer / instant pot, covered, on medium.

SERVE IT WITH: To make this a complete meal, serve with creamy cucumber salad.

PER SERVING

calories: 432 | fat: 19.2g | total carbs: 2.7g | fiber: 0.5g | protein: 61.8g

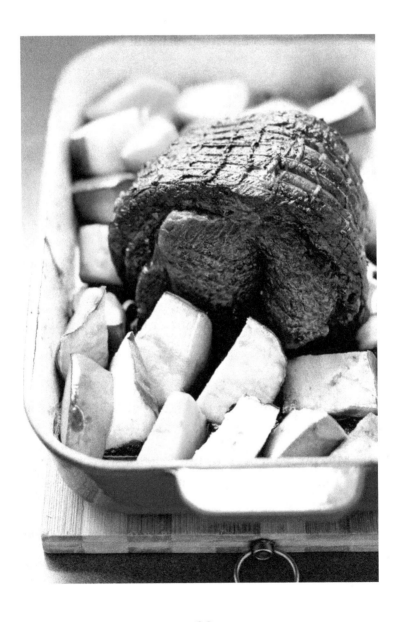

Spicy Lamb Meat

Macros: Fat 62% | Protein 33% | Carbs 5%

Prep time: 5 minutes | Cook time: 20 minutes | Serves 4

This is a versatile dish with low-carb content. It is keto-approved and easy to cook. It is the perfect dish to stay healthy.

- 1 tablespoon minced garlic
- 1 tablespoon minced ginger
- 2 tablespoons butter
- 1 cup chopped onions
- ½ teaspoon turmeric powder
- ½ teaspoon cayenne pepper
- ½ teaspoon ground coriander
- 1½ teaspoon cumin powder 1 teaspoon salt
- 1 pound (454 g) ground lamb meat

In a nonstick skillet, add garlic, ginger, butter, and onions and mix well. Sauté for approximately 3 minutes and add the turmeric powder, cayenne pepper, coriander, cumin powder, salt and lamb meat.

Put the lid on and cook on medium-high heat for 20 minutes until the lamb meat is cooked through.

Transfer into a serving platter to cool before serving.

STORAGE: Store in an airtight container in the refrigerator for up to 4 days.

REHEAT: Microwave, covered, until the desired temperature is reached or reheat in a frying pan or air fryer / instant pot, covered, on medium.

SERVE IT WITH: To make this a complete meal, serve with cabbage and egg salad.

PER SERVING

calories: 291 | fat: 20.1g | total carbs: 4.4g | fiber: 0.8g | protein: 23.8g

Keto Maui Wowie Shrimp

Macros: Fat 68% | Protein 31% | Carbs 1%

Prep time: 15 minutes | Cook time: 10 minutes | Serves 6

A quick, easy, and delicious grilled shrimp recipe. These Maui wowie shrimp will be on your table in under 20 minutes, which makes them excellent for a busy night!

- 1tablespoon olive oil
- 2 pounds (907 g) medium-sized raw shrimp, peeled and deveined
- ¼ teaspoon garlic salt
- Freshly ground pepper, to taste
- 1 cup keto-friendly mayonnaise 1 large lemon, sliced

SPECIAL EQUIPMENT:

Bamboo skewers, soaked for at least 30 minutes

Preheat the grill to medium heat and grease the grill grates lightly with olive oil.

Thread 3 to 4 shrimp onto the bamboo skewers. Make sure the shrimp are all in the same direction.

Season the shrimp with salt and pepper on both sides.

Using a silicone brush, generously coat the shrimp with mayonnaise on both sides.

Place the shrimp on the preheated grill, cook for about 5 minutes per side, or wait until the shrimp is pink and opaque.

Transfer the shrimp to a plate and serve with lemon slices.

STORAGE: Store in an airtight container in the fridge for up to 4 days or in the freezer for up to 1 month.

REHEAT: Microwave, covered, until the desired temperature is reached or reheat in a frying pan or air fryer/instant pot, covered, on medium.

SERVE IT WITH: This dish goes well with warm kale salad, cauliflower rice, or zucchini noodles.

PER SERVING

calories: 401 | fat: 30.5g | total carbs: 0.8g | fiber: 0g | protein: 30.8g

Grilled Red Lobster Tails

Macros: Fat 43% | Protein 56% | Carbs 1%

Prep time:15 minutes | Cook time: 12 minutes | Serves 2

Treat your family and friends to this delicious and easy version of grilled red lobster tails! This recipe uses a special blend of lemon, garlic, and paprika, which perfectly complements the lobsters' sweetness.

- 1 tablespoon freshly squeezed lemon juice
- ½ cup extra virgin olive oil
- ½ tablespoon salt Pinch of garlic powder
- ½ tablespoon paprika Pinch of white pepper
- 2 (10-ounce / 284-g) red lobster tails
- 1 teaspoon olive oil, for greasing the grill grates

Preheat the grill to high heat.

In a bowl, whisk together the lemon juice, olive oil, salt, garlic powder, paprika, and white pepper.

Using a large knife, cut open lobster tails and slice lengthwise. Brush the flesh side of lobster tail with the marinade.

Lightly grease the grill grates with olive oil. Place the tails on the preheated grill, flesh-side down. Grill for about 10 minutes, flipping once, or until the lobster is opaque. Frequently baste tails with the marinade.

Let cool for 5 minutes before serving.

STORAGE: Place lobster tails in an airtight container and store in the fridge for up to three days.

REHEAT: Microwave, covered, until the desired temperature is reached or reheat in an air fryer or instant pot, covered, on medium.

SERVE IT WITH: This dish goes well with warm kale salad, cauliflower rice, or zucchini noodles.

PER SERVING

calories: 416 | fat: 20.1g | total carbs: 1.7g | fiber: 0.7g | protein: 57.8g

Keto Taco Fishbowl

Macros: Fat 77% | Protein 13% | Carbs 10%

Prep time: 5 minutes | Cook time: 10 minutes | Serves 4

Are you tired of eating daily repeated dishes? Just try to make keto taco fishbowl yourself. It doesn't take much time to be prepared. This recipe is very simple to be prepared and it's also rich in the ingredients.

DRESSING:

- ½ cup keto-friendly mayonnaise 2 tablespoons lime juice
- 1 teaspoon hot sauce
- ½ teaspoon garlic powder
- Salt and freshly ground black pepper, to taste

MAIN MEAL:

- ½ pound (227 g) green cabbage or red cabbage
- ½ yellow onion
- 1 tomato
- 1 avocado
- Salt and ground black pepper, to taste
- 3 tablespoons olive oil, divided
- 10 ounces (284 g) white fish, patted dry
- 1 tablespoon Tex-Mex seasoning
- Fresh cilantro, for garnish
- Lime, for garnish

In a bowl, mix the ingredients for the dressing before frying the fish, so the flavors have time to develop. Allow to sit at room temperature or keep in the refrigerator.

With a sharp knife or mandolin, shred or slice all vegetables finely except the avocado. Split the avocado in half and remove the pit. Slice the avocado thinly and using a spoon to scoop avocado slices out of the skin. Season the vegetables and avocado slices with salt and pepper on a plate, then drizzle with 2 tablespoons olive oil. Toss well and set aside.

Rub both sides of white fish with salt, pepper, and Tex-Mex seasoning.

In a skillet, add the remaining olive oil. Fry the fish in olive oil over medium heat for 3 to 4 minutes on both sides, or until the fish flakes easily with a fork.

Transfer the vegetable mixture to a serving bowl. Top with the fish and pour over the dressing. Garnish with fresh cilantro and lime before serving.

STORAGE: Store the leftovers in an airtight container in the fridge for up to 3 days.

REHEAT: Wrap the fish in a foil with a little olive oil to keep it moist and then put it into the oven at about 200°F (93°C) for 5 to 7 minutes.

SERVE IT WITH: To make this a complete meal, serve it with mushroom soup or vegetable roasted salad.

PER SERVING

calories: 489 | fat: 42.9g | total carbs: 14.2g | fiber: 5.6g | protein: 15.1g

Low Carb Poached Eggs with Tuna Salad

Macros: Fat 68% | Protein 27% | Carbs 5%

Prep time: 10 minutes | Cook time: 10 minutes | Serves 2

When you make this colorful recipe, don't forget to take a shot and post it to your Instagram to let your friends know how gorgeous you are! Low-carb poached eggs with tuna salad is an elegant dish to go with any main meal.

TUNA SALAD:

- 4 ounces (113 g) tuna in olive oil, rinsed and drained
- ⅓ cup chopped celery stalks
- ½ red onion
- ½ cup mayonnaise, keto-friendly
- 1 teaspoon Dijon mustard
- Juice and zest of ½ lemon
- Salt and freshly ground black pepper, to taste

POACHED EGGS:

- 4 eggs
- 1 teaspoon salt
- 2 teaspoons white wine vinegar or white vinegar
- 2 tablespoons olive oil
- 2 ounces (57 g) leafy greens or lettuce
- 2 ounces (57 g) cherry tomatoes, chopped

Chop the tuna and mix it in a bowl with the other ingredients for the salad. You can make it ahead of time and keep it in the refrigerator. The flavor will enhance with time.

Bring a pot of water to a boil over medium heat. Add the vinegar and salt, then stir the water in circles to create a swirl using a spoon. Crack the eggs into the pot, one at a time.

Let simmer for 3 minutes and use a slotted spoon to remove it from the water.

Transfer the eggs to the bowl of tuna salad and drizzle with olive oil.

Gently toss until everything is combined.

Serve them with leafy greens and cherry tomatoes on the side.

STORAGE: Store in an airtight container in the fridge for up to 3 days.

REHEAT: Microwave, covered, until the desired temperature is reached or reheat in a frying pan or air fryer / instant pot, covered, on medium.

PER SERVING

calories: 534 | fat: 40.5g | total carbs: 7.2g | fiber: 1.4g | protein: 34.0g

Smoked Salmon and Lettuce Bites

Macros: Fat 73% | Protein 20% | Carbs 7%

Prep time: 20 minutes | Cook time: 0 minutes | Serves 6

After finishing your work with relaxation and let your little brother prepare this dish for the whole family. How is that! Yes, this is the smoked salmon bites that need no oven to be prepared. Simple, speedy, and suitable for any main dish.

- 7 ounces (198 g) smoked salmon, cut into small pieces
- 8 ounces (227 g) cream cheese
- ⅓ tablespoon mayonnaise, keto-friendly
- 4 tablespoons chopped fresh dill or fresh chives
- ½ lemon, zested
- ¼ teaspoon ground black pepper
- 2 ounces (57 g) lettuce, for serving

Add the cream cheese, mayonnaise, fresh dill, lemon zest, and pepper in a bowl. Stir to combine well.

Lay the lettuce on a clean work surface. Top with the salmon pieces and pour the cream cheese mixture over. Serve immediately.

STORAGE: Store in an airtight container in the fridge for up to 3 days.

REHEAT: Microwave the salmon, covered, until the desired temperature is reached or reheat in a frying pan or air fryer / instant pot, covered, on medium.

SERVE IT WITH: You can serve with thinly sliced and toasted low-carb keto bread or crunchy vegetables.

PER SERVING

calories: 179 | fat: 15.0g | total carbs: 3.3g | fiber: 1.1g | protein: 8.6g

Cauliflower Hash with Poblano Peppers

Macros: Fat: 88% | Protein: 8% | Carb: 4%

Prep time: 10 minutes | Cook time: 15 minutes | Serves 4

The dish gives you a variety of options to have some makeover. Try any other dairy products of your choice to make it special. Serving crumbled feta along with the baked peppers will be a fantastic option to make the dish tasty. If you want to make the salad more colorful, go for different colored peppers, and maintain the spiciness as per your preference.

- ½ cup keto-friendly mayonnaise
- 1 teaspoon garlic powder
- 1 pound (454 g) shredded cauliflower
- 3 ounces (85 g) butter, melted
- Salt and freshly ground black pepper, to taste
- 1 teaspoon virgin olive oil
- 3 ounces (85 g) poblano peppers
- 4 eggs

In a small bowl, combine the mayonnaise and garlic powder and set aside.

In a food processor, grate the cauliflower with the stem.

In a large skillet, fry the grated cauliflower in melted butter. Sprinkle pepper and salt to taste. Transfer to a plate. Set aside until ready to serve.

Apply the olive oil on the poblano peppers and fry in the skillet until blistered. Remove from the skillet and set aside.

Break the eggs in the skillet and fry.for 2 minutes on each side Season with pepper and salt.

Serve the fried eggs with cauliflower hash and fried poblanos.

STORAGE: Store in an airtight container in the fridge for up to 3 days.

SERVE IT WITH: It can use as a breakfast or brunch. Alternatively, it can serve as a ketogenic side dish.

PER SERVING

calories: 450 | fat: 43.9g | total carbs: 4.7g | fiber: 3.0g | protein: 8.7g

Lemony Coleslaw

Macros: Fat: 92% | Protein: 2% | Carb: 6%

Prep time: 5 minutes | Cook time: 10 minutes | Serves 4

Coleslaw is a yummy side dish, and here I am, presenting a ketogenic coleslaw that will go easy with health-conscious people. It is ideal for serving along with a BBQ dish or a family get together. The low-calorie dish is easy to make, and in about 10 minutes, you are ready with the dish. The process simply matches the restaurant type coleslaw makes your friend awestruck. I recommend people to use mayonnaise to meet the keto restrictions. Make some experiments to change the traditional taste. You can roast the fennel seeds and mix with the coleslaw for having an improved taste.

- 8 ounces (227 g) fresh cabbage, cored
- ½ lemon juice extract
- 1 teaspoon salt
- ⅛ teaspoon ground black pepper
- ½ cup keto-friendly mayonnaise
- 1 tablespoon Dijon mustard
- ⅛ teaspoon fennel seeds

Grate the cabbage in a food processor. Put the grated cabbage in a medium bowl. Drizzle with the lemon juice, and sprinkle salt and pepper over it.

Toss the cabbage to coat well. Let it sit for about 10 minutes until it becomes soft. Drain out excess liquid.

Add the mayonnaise and mustard and combine it well.

Sprinkle with fennel seeds and serve.

STORAGE: Refrigerate the coleslaw in a tight container for later use. It can ideally use for 3 to 4 days if stored well.

SERVE IT WITH: It is an ideal choice if served along with BBQ, roasted / baked chicken, meat, or fish.

PER SERVING

calories: 209 | fat: 21.7g | total carbs: 3.1g | fiber: 2.4g | protein: 1.3g

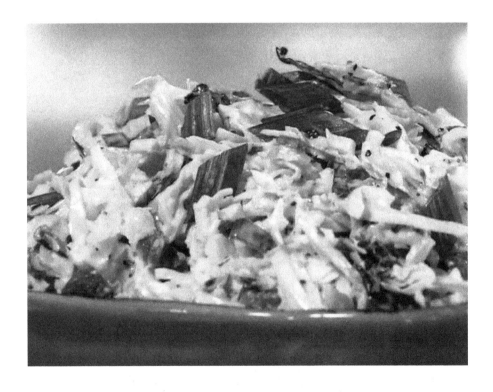

Guacamole

Macros: Fat: 86% | Protein: 6% | Carb: 8%

Prep time: 15 minutes | Cook time: 0 minutes | Serves 4

Enjoy the mashed delicacy of avocadoes, combined with grated onion, lime juice, and spices. The salad is quick to make and easy to make some alteration. Consider adding salsa and sour cream along with the ingredients to augment the taste. The calorie content justifies its ketogenic effect.

- 2 ripe avocados
- ½ lime, juice extracted
- ½ white onion, finely grated
- 1 tomato, diced
- 4 tablespoons garden-fresh cilantro, finely chopped
- 1 clove garlic, finely grated
- 2 tablespoons virgin olive oil
- ¼ teaspoon ground pepper
- ¼ teaspoon salt

Peel the avocados and mash it in a medium bowl using a fork.

Combine it with lime juice, grated onion, tomato, cilantro, minced garlic, and olive oil.

Add pepper and salt as per your taste and combine well before serving.

STORAGE: Store in an airtight container in the fridge for 4 to 5 days.

SERVE IT WITH: Combine well with fried fish, roasted chicken, and meat.

PER SERVING

calories: 238 | fat: 22.4g | total carbs: 5.1g | fiber: 3.2g | protein: 3.4g

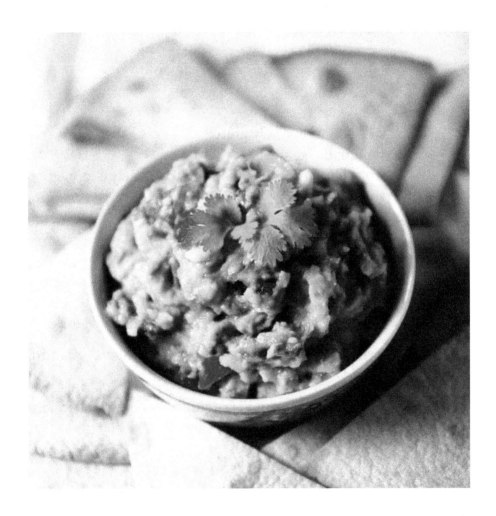

Vegetables Tricolor

Macros: Fat: 88% | Protein: 9% | Carb: 3%

Prep time: 10 minutes | Cook time: 20 minutes | Serves 6

The colorful salad is something special everybody loves to have. It is a low- carb keto diet with a focus on the delicacy quotient. With a quick preparation, you can complete the cooking within 20 minutes in a flavor-rich aroma. For maintaining tricolor, the salad uses fresh Brussels sprouts, cherry tomatoes, and mushrooms. The grilled salad will be a trendsetter and relishing side dish delicacy.

- 1 pound (454 g) Brussels sprouts
- 8 ounces (227 g) mushrooms
- 8 ounces (227 g) cherry tomatoes
- ½ cup olive oil
- 1 teaspoon salt
- ½ teaspoon ground pepper
- 1 teaspoon dried thyme

Preheat the oven to 400°F (205°C).

Rinse and chop all the vegetables in equal size. Put the chopped vegetables in a medium bowl. Add olive oil, salt, pepper, dried thyme, and mix well.

Line a parchment paper in a baking dish and spread the vegetable in it.

Roast the vegetable in the preheated oven for about 20 minutes or until the vegetable becomes soft, and the color looks good.

Remove them from the oven and serve.

STORAGE: After settling the heat, the dish can refrigerate in a tight container for an extended shelve life. In normal condition, you will have a shelve life of 5 days, if refrigerated properly.

SERVE IT WITH: It is an ideal dish to serve along with a dipping sauce. You can add any vegetable of choice and spices to give a personal touch. It is a perfect side dish for fried chicken, fish, and meat.

PER SERVING

calories: 188 | fat: 18.3g | total carbs: 6.1g | fiber: 4.3g | protein: 4.4g

Zucchini and Walnut Salad

Macros: Fat: 92% | Protein: 7% | Carb: 1%

Prep time: 20 minutes | Cook time: 15 minutes | Serves 4

Dressings are the key ingredients that make any salad delicious. Design the dressing menu as the way you wish and give a surprise to your guests. I have divided the zucchini and walnut salad into two sections, starting with the salad and followed by the dressing. You will fall in love with the crunchy and nutty taste of roasted zucchinis.

FOR DRESSING:

- ¾ cup keto-friendly mayonnaise
- 2 tablespoons virgin olive oil
- 2 teaspoons lemon juice
- 1 tablespoon minced clove garlic
- ¼ teaspoon chili powder
- ¼ teaspoon salt

FOR SALAD:

- 4 ounces (113 g) arugula lettuce
- ¼ cup sliced fresh chives
- 1 head Romaine lettuce
- 2 zucchinis
- 1 tablespoon virgin olive oil
- ¼ teaspoon salt
- ½ teaspoon ground pepper
- 3½ ounces (99 g) chopped walnuts

Make the dressing: In a medium bowl, combine all the dressing ingredients. Set aside.

Make the salad: Trim the ends of the vegetables if required and cut them into uniform size. In a large bowl, combine the sliced arugula, chives, and Romaine lettuce.

Cut the zucchini in lengthwise and remove the seeds. Then cut the zucchini splits into halves making it into half-inch pieces.

In a large frying pan, pour olive oil and bring to medium heat. When the oil becomes hot, put zucchini into the pan, sprinkle salt and pepper to season. Sauté until the zucchini pieces become brown but remain firm.

Transfer the cooked zucchini pieces into the salad bowl and combine them gently.

Roast the nuts in the frying pan for 7 minutes or until browned evenly.

Sprinkle with pepper and salt. Transfer the nuts onto the salad and mix.

Pour the dressing over the salad and combine gently before serving.

STORAGE: Ideally, you can keep the salad refrigerated for 5 days in an airtight container. Scoop out only what you want to serve 15 minutes before serving.

SERVE IT WITH: The salad goes well with roasted or grilled chicken, fish, and meat. There is no limit for experimenting, as long it can make you confident.

PER SERVING

calories: 565 | fat: 58.1g | total carbs: 8.4g | fiber: 6.9g | protein: 9.3g

Stewed Meat and Pumpkin

Macros: Fat 59% | Protein 26% | Carbs 15%

Prep time: 15 minutes | Cook time: 44 minutes | Serves 6

Satisfy your meat desires while on a keto diet with the delicious stewed meat and pumpkin. The recipe is enriched with a variety of ingredients for body nourishment. You can prepare this meal for lunch or dinner.

- 1 tablespoon olive oil
- ½ cup chopped onion
- 1 minced garlic clove
- 2 pounds (907 g) chopped pork stew meat
- ½ cup dry white wine
- 1 cup pumpkin purée
- 1 tablespoon butter
- ¼ cup stevia
- ¼ teaspoon cardamom powder
- 2 cups water
- 2 cups chicken stock
- Salt and freshly ground black pepper, to taste
- 1 teaspoon lemon juice

In a large saucepan, melt the olive oil then fry the onions until translucent, for about 3 minutes.

Add the garlic and cook until soft, about 1 minute.

Add the pork and cook for about 6 minutes until browned.

Pour in the white wine and cook for 1 minute more.

Add the pumpkin purée, butter, stevia, cardamom powder, water, and chicken stock. Allow to boil for 5 minutes.

Cover and reduce the heat to low. Simmer for 30 minutes. Season as needed with salt and pepper to taste.

Mix in the lemon juice, then transfer to serving bowls and serve.

STORAGE: Store in an airtight container in the fridge for up to 1 week

REHEAT: Microwave, covered, until the desired temperature is reached or reheat in a frying pan or instant pot, covered, on medium.

SERVE IT WITH: To make this a complete meal, serve the stewed meat and pumpkin with Mexican-style cauliflower rice.

PER SERVING

calories: 315 | fat: 11.3g | total carbs: 6.6g | fiber: 0.3g | protein: 47.1g

Bay Scallop and Bacon Chowder

Macros: Fat 69% | Protein 20% | Carbs 11%

Prep time: 35 minutes | Cook time: 25 minutes | Serves 6

With only a handful of ingredients, this soup is simple to throw together, and the flavors shine on their own, especially the bay scallops, which have a magical way of transforming any dish it is in. The fare is a tasty way to enjoy the sweet, tender, and creamy bay scallops. And the daikon radish is a delicious and perfect vegetable in making a keto-friendly soup. So if you want something comforting, yet light and quick, then this bay scallop chowder is the one for you.

- 1 tablespoon butter
- 4 slices bacon chopped
- 3 cups chopped daikon radish
- 1 medium onion chopped
- 2½ cups chicken stock
- ½ teaspoon dried thyme
- Salt and freshly ground black pepper, to taste
- 1 pound (454 g) bay scallops
- 2 cups heavy cream

Heat a large saucepan over medium heat and melt the butter.

Add the bacon and fry until crisp. Then add the daikon radish and onion to it and cook for 4 minutes.

Pour the chicken stock and allow it to simmer for 7 minutes.

Sprinkle with thyme, pepper, and salt. Mix to combine well.

Add bay scallops and heavy cream to the soup and simmer for further 5 minutes. Stir to combine well.

Remove the saucepan from the heat and serve the chowder hot in serving bowls.

STORAGE: Store in an airtight container in the refrigerator for up to 4 days.

REHEAT: Microwave, covered, until the desired temperature is reached or reheat in an instant pot, covered, on medium.

SERVE IT WITH: To make this a complete meal, serve the soup along with baked beef rolls. If you prefer a healthier side dish, then have it with kale Caesar salad.

PER SERVING

calories: 400 | fat: 30.9g | total carbs: 11.5g | sugars: 1.4g | protein: 20.5g

Easy Brazilian Shrimp Stew (Moqueca De Camaroes)

Macros: Fat 60% | Protein 33% | Carbs 7%

Prep time: 25 minutes | Cook time: 20 minutes | Serves 6

Indulge in this simple yet outrageously scrumptious stew, and you will find yourself in heaven. Spiked with the flavors of lime, cilantro, and coconut, the soup is light and full of fresh taste. The soup has a luxurious texture from the coconut milk while having a fiery heat and tropical tang from the seasonings. If possible, try to get hold of red palm oil, which can give the soup a distinctive signature floral note. In Brazil, the stew is a must-have at any Latin table, especially on Easter.

- ¼ cup olive oil
- 1 garlic clove, minced
- ¼ cup onions, diced
- 1(14-ounce / 397-g) can diced tomatoes with chilies
- ¼ cup red pepper, roasted and diced
- ¼ cup fresh cilantro, chopped plus extra for garnish
- 1½ pounds (680 g) raw shrimp, peeled and deveined
- 1 cup unsweetened coconut milk
- 2 tablespoons Sriracha hot sauce
- Salt and freshly ground black pepper, to taste
- 2 tablespoons lemon juice
- Fresh cilantro, for garnish

Start by adding olive oil to a heated medium saucepan and then spoon in the garlic and onion.

Sauté the onion-garlic mixture for 2 minutes and stir in tomatoes, pepper, cilantro, and shrimp.

Sauté for 4 minutes or until the shrimp is opaque. Pour coconut milk and Sriracha sauce over it.

Simmer the soup for 4 minutes and add pepper, salt, and lime juice. Do not bring the soup to a boil.

Top it with the fresh cilantro and transfer to soup bowls to serve.

STORAGE: Store in an airtight container in the refrigerator for up to 3 days or the freezer for up to 2 months.

REHEAT: Microwave, covered, until the desired temperature is reached or reheat in an instant pot, covered, on medium.

SERVE IT WITH: To make this a complete meal, you can spoon the delicious stew over hot steamed cauliflower rice. Or you can serve it with gluten-free bread of your choice.

PER SERVING

calories: 305 | fat: 20.2g | total carbs: 7.0g | fiber: 1.2g | protein: 24.9g

Creamy Crockpot Chicken Stew

Macros: Fat 50% | Protein 40% | Carbs 10%

Prep time: 5 minutes | Cook time: 4 hours | Serves 6

Here is an excellent chicken stew recipe that is so hearty and healthy, which is ideal for chilly nights. In fact, there is nothing more cozy and comforting than this crockpot chicken stew. And the radish is a delicious and perfect vegetable in making a keto-friendly soup. With just a few minutes of prep, you can make this satisfying classic comfort food dinner that is a meal unto itself as it is loaded with protein and vegetables. For a depth of flavor, you can pour over some dry red wine.

- 1.7 pounds (794 g) skinless and deboned chicken thighs, diced into 1-inch pieces
- ½ teaspoon dried oregano
- ½ onion, diced
- ½ teaspoon dried rosemary
- 2 cups chicken stock
- ½ cup radish, peeled and finely diced
- 2 celery sticks, diced
- 3garlic cloves, minced
- ¼ teaspoon dried thyme
- Salt and black pepper, to taste
- ½ cup heavy cream
- ½ teaspoon xanthan gum
- 1 cup fresh spinach

In the crockpot, add the chicken thighs, oregano, onion, rosemary, chicken stock, radish, celery, garlic, and thyme. Stir to combine well.

Press the 'low' heat button and cook for 4 hours.

Sprinkle salt and pepper over the chicken mixture and then add heavy cream, xanthan gum, and spinach.

Cook further for 9 minutes while stirring it continuously.

Transfer the stew from the crockpot to the serving bowl and serve it hot.

STORAGE: Store in an airtight container in the refrigerator for up to 3 days or the freezer for up to 3 months.

REHEAT: Microwave, covered, until the desired temperature is reached or reheat in a crockpot or instant pot, covered, on low.

SERVE IT WITH: To make this a complete meal, you can have the stew along with a veggie salad and roasted chicken thighs.

PER SERVING

calories: 227 | fat: 10.2g | total carbs: 5.8g | fiber: 0.6g | protein: 28.8g

Keto Beef Stew

Macros: Fat 58% | Protein 37% | Carbs 5%

Prep time: 10 minutes | Cook time: 1 hour | Serves 4

Have you ever made something so rich, so savory, that it makes you go weak in the knees? This stew with fork-tender beef does that to me. It is that kind of comfort food which you would want to have all winter long. On top, the stew is thick, hearty and full of amazing classic flavor which tastes so better the next day.

- 1 tablespoon coconut oil
- 1 pound (454 g) beef short rib
- ¼ teaspoon pink salt
- ¼ teaspoon freshly ground black pepper
- 4 cloves garlic, minced
- 1 tablespoon butter
- ¾ cup sliced onions
- 2 cups beef broth
- ½ teaspoon xanthan gum
- ¾ cup radishes

Take a large saucepan and heat it over medium-high heat. Add the coconut oil and beef short ribs to it.

Apply pink salt and pepper over the ribs. Sear the meat for 3 minutes per side or until browned.

Then stir in the garlic, butter, and onion. Continue cooking for a further 3 minutes.

Pour the beef broth along with the xanthan gum and bring the mixture to a boil.

Allow it to simmer for 25 minutes and stir in the radishes.

Cook for further 25 minutes while stirring it continuously.

Transfer the stew from the saucepan to the serving bowl. Enjoy it hot.

STORAGE: Store in an airtight container in the refrigerator for up to 3 days or the freezer for up to 3 months.

REHEAT: Microwave, covered, until the desired temperature is reached or reheat in a pan / instant pot, covered, on low.

SERVE IT WITH: To make this a complete meal, you can serve it along with mashed cauliflower or roasted Brussels sprouts.

PER SERVING

calories: 262 | fat: 16.8g | total carbs: 3.9g | fiber: 0.1g | protein: 24.8g

Zesty Double Beef Stew

Macros: Fat 27% | Protein 65% | Carbs 8%

Prep time: 10 minutes | Cook time: 8 hours | Serves 6

A few simple ingredients make this a sumptuous stew. It has the perfect combination of tender beef and spicy seasonings that is so full of flavor. You are sure to be blown away by the taste. And if you are ready to up the spice level still more, you can even add a spoon of red pepper flakes to the stew.

- 1½ pounds (680 g) stew beef
- 1 tablespoon Lea & Perrins Worcestershire sauce
- 1 (14½-ounce / 411-g) can chili-ready diced tomatoes
- 2 teaspoons Sriracha hot sauce
- 1 tablespoon chili mix
- 1 cup beef broth
- Salt, to taste

In the crockpot, place the stew beef, Worcestershire sauce, diced tomatoes, hot sauce, chili mix, beef broth, and salt. Mix well.

Turn the crockpot on high power for 6 hours. Then pull apart the meat in the crockpot with a fork.

Sprinkle with more salt if needed and cook for further 2 hours on low heat.

Transfer the stew from the crockpot to the serving bowl. Enjoy it hot.

STORAGE: Store in an airtight container in the refrigerator for up to 3 days or the freezer for up to 3 months.

REHEAT: Microwave, covered, until the desired temperature is reached or reheat in a pan / instant pot, covered, on low.

SERVE IT WITH: To make this a complete meal, you can pair it with cauliflower rice.

PER SERVING

calories: 161 | fat: 4.9g | total carbs: 3.8g | fiber: 0.5g | protein: 26.0g

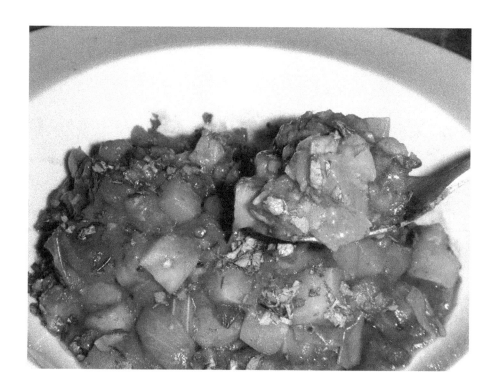

Rich Beef Stew with Dumpling

Macros: Fat 42% | Protein 46% | Carbs 12%

Prep time: 10 minutes | Cook time: 4 hours | Serves 8

Comforting, cozy, and warming, this highly indulgent fare is a delightfully tender stew with melt in your mouth tender beef pieces. And the daikon radish is a delicious and perfect vegetable in making a keto-friendly soup. The flavor explosion when you take the first bite is so good and indisputable. Though I eat this by itself, if you want to make, you can replace the dumplings to mashed cauliflower.

- 2 tablespoons olive oil, divided
- 2 pounds (907 g) stew beef
- 1 red onion, chopped
- 1 daikon radish, chopped
- 3½ ounces (99-g) pumpkin, chopped
- 3 sprigs of fresh rosemary
- 3 bay leaves
- 2 cloves garlic, minced
- ½ cup dry red wine
- 2 cups beef stock
- ¾ teaspoon sea salt
- ¼ teaspoon black pepper

DUMPLINGS:

- ¾ cup almond flour
- ⅓ cup sesame seed flour 1 tablespoon fresh thyme
- 1 tablespoon psyllium husk powder
- 1 cup water, boiling
- ¼ cup coconut flour

- 1½ teaspoons gluten-free baking powder
- 1 tablespoon chopped rosemary
- ¼ teaspoon of sea salt 1 pinch black pepper
- 3 large egg whites
- 1 large beaten egg
- 1 teaspoon fresh lemon zest, for garnish
- Fresh parsley, for garnish

Preheat the oven to 325°F (160°C).

Heat a large saucepan over medium heat and place 1 tablespoon of olive oil and beef in it.

Sear the meat for 4 minutes on each side or until browned. Transfer to a paper-lined plate.

Pour the remaining oil to it along with onion, radish, and pumpkin.

Sauté the vegetables for 8 minutes and add rosemary, bay leaves, garlic, and browned meat.

Cook for a further 2 minutes and pour the wine. Lower the heat and continue cooking for an additional 4 minutes.

Stir in the stock, salt, and pepper. Mix well and allow it to boil. Pour the mixture to the baking dish.

Roast the mixture for 3 hours. Remove from the oven and increase the temperature of the oven to 350°F (180°C).

In the meantime, combine almond flour, sesame seed flour, thyme, husk powder, water, coconut flour, baking powder, rosemary, salt, pepper, egg whites and egg. Make dumplings out of this dough.

Keep the dumplings in greased cupcake tins and bake in the oven for 23 minutes.

Flip with a spoon and bake for another 4 minutes.

Gently place the dumplings into the stew and gently stir.

Serve in bowls and enjoy it hot. Garnish with lemon zest and parsley.

STORAGE: Store in an airtight container in the refrigerator for up to 3 days. If you are planning to freeze, make, and add the dumplings on day before.

REHEAT: Microwave, covered, until the desired temperature is reached or reheat in a pan / instant pot, covered, on low.

SERVE IT WITH: To make this a complete meal, you can serve it with a cherry tomato and mushroom salad and fried pork chop.

PER SERVING

calories: 282 | fat: 10.8g | total carbs: 9.8g | fiber: 1.2g | protein: 32.2g

Mexican-Style Scrambled Eggs

Macros: Fat 68% | Protein 24% | Carbs 7%

Prep time: 5 minutes | Cook time: 10 minutes | Serves 4

Prepare this dish for your breakfast. Filled with the flavorful eggs, tomatoes, jalapeños, and scallions, you will have wonderful breakfast moments to spice up your day.

- 1 ounce (28 g) butter
- 1 chopped tomato
- 1chopped scallion
- 2chopped pickled jalapeños pepper
- 6 eggs
- Salt and freshly ground black pepper, to taste
- 3 ounces (85 g) shredded cheese

Put the butter in a medium pan over medium-high heat to melt.

Add the tomatoes, scallions, and jalapeños, then cook for 4 minutes until tender.

Beat the eggs in a small bowl, then add to the pan. Cook as you scramble for 2 minutes.

Sprinkle with the pepper, cheese, and salt. Stir well and serve warm.

STORAGE: Store in an airtight container in the fridge for up to 4 days.

REHEAT: Microwave, covered, until the desired temperature is reached or reheat in a frying pan, covered, on medium.

SERVE IT WITH: To makv this a complete meal, serve the eggs with crisp lettuce, avocados, and a dressing to add taste.

PER SERVING

calories: 216 | fat: 16.7g | total carbs: 4.3g | fiber: 0.7g | protein: 12.2g

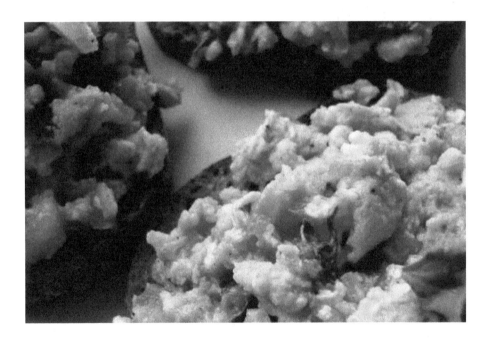

Fluffy Western Omelet

Macros: Fat 73% | Protein 23% | Carbs 4%

Prep time: 5 minutes | Cook time: 25 minutes | Serves 2

Enjoy the fluffy filled with cheesy egg goodness omelet. This keto meal will fulfill our choices for dinner, lunch, or even breakfast. Filled with tasty flavors from bell pepper, ham, and onion, you will love it.

- 2 tablespoons heavy whipping cream or sour cream
- 6 eggs
- Salt and freshly ground pepper, to taste
- 3 ounces (85 g) shredded cheese
- 2 ounces (57 g) butter
- ½ chopped green bell pepper
- 5 ounces (142 g) diced smoked deli ham
- ½ chopped yellow onion

Whisk the cream and eggs in a bowl until fluffy, then add the pepper and salt. Stir well.

Mix in half of the shredded cheese and set aside.

In a large pan, melt the butter over medium heat. Add the peppers, ham, and onions and fry for 5 minutes. Pour in the egg mixture and cook until it is almost firm, making sure not to burn the edges.

Reduce the heat to low, then top with the remaining cheese.

Transfer to a plate and slice in half before serving.

STORAGE: Store in an airtight container in the fridge for up to 4 days. It is not recommended to freeze.

REHEAT: Microwave, covered, until the desired temperature is reached or reheat in a frying pan, covered, on medium.

SERVE IT WITH: To make this a complete meal, serve the omelet with your preferred green salad. The omelet also goes well with jalapeños and low-carb Sriracha sauce.

PER SERVING

calories: 872 | fat: 71.3g | total carbs: 10.7g | fiber: 0.5g | protein: 46.9g

Homemade Cheddar Crackers

Macros: Fat: 67% | Protein: 29% | Carbs: 4%

Prep time: 15 minutes | Cook time: 20 minutes | Serves 4

One of the easy to make crackers that are addicting! These homemade crackers are super cheesy with a delicious kick.

- 1 cup almond flour
- ½ cup Cheddar cheese, shredded finely
- 1 tablespoon nutritional yeast
- ¼ teaspoon baking soda
- ¼ teaspoon garlic powder
- ¼ teaspoon sea salt
- 2 teaspoons olive oil
- 1 egg
- Olive oil spray

Preheat your oven to 350°F (180°C) and line a baking sheet with parchment paper. Lightly grease two parchment papers with olive oil spray and set them aside.

In a large mixing bowl, add the almond flour, Cheddar cheese, nutritional yeast, baking soda, garlic powder, and salt and mix well. In a separate bowl, place the oil and egg, then beat until well combined. Add the egg mixture into the flour mixture bowl and with a wooden spoon, mix well until a dough ball forms.

On a flat work surface, knead the dough for 1 to 2 minutes with your hands. Arrange 1 greased parchment paper onto the work surface. Place the dough ball onto the greased parchment paper and with your hands, then press into a disk. Arrange another greased parchment paper on top of dough, then roll it into a

9×12-inch (⅛-inch thick) rectangle with a rolling pin. With a pizza cutter, cut the edges of the dough into an even rectangle. Now, cut the dough into 1½×1½-inch columns and rows. Arrange the crackers onto the prepared baking sheet. Bake for about 15 to 20 minutes or until crispy.

Remove from the oven to a wire rack to cool completely before serving.

STORAGE: Place the crackers in an airtight container and store at room temperature for up to 1 week.

SERVE IT WITH: Spread a thin layer of cream cheese over crackers and top with crispy bacon bits before serving.

PER SERVING

calories: 184 | fat: 13.8g | total carbs: 1.8g | fiber: 0.3g | protein: 7.2g

Watercress and Arugula Turkey Salad

Macros: Fat 68% | Protein 27% | Carbs 5%

Prep time: 12 minutes | Cook time: 13 minutes | Serves 4

The turkey transforms this salad into a classic light dinner that is irresistibly delicious and that will leave everyone asking for more.

DRESSING:

- 1 tablespoon xylitol
- 2 tablespoons lime juice
- 1 tablespoon Dijon mustard
- 1 red onion, chopped
- 1¾ cups raspberries, divided
- 5 tablespoons olive oil, divided
- ¼ cup water
- Salt and freshly ground black pepper, to taste

SALAD :

- 1 pound (454 g) boneless turkey breast, slice in half 1 cup watercress
- 1 cup arugula
- 4 ounces (113 g) goat cheese, crumbled
- ½ cup walnuts, halved

Make the dressing: Add xylitol, lime juice, Dijon mustard, onion, 1 cup of raspberries, 3 tablespoons olive oil, water, salt, and pepper in a high- powered blender. Pulse until smooth.

Strain the liquid from the mixture in a mixing bowl and set aside.

On a flat work surface, generously season the turkey breasts with salt and pepper.

Heat a saucepan over medium heat, then coat the bottom with 2 tablespoons olive oil. Place the turkey in the heated saucepan, skin-side down. Cook the turkey for 8 minutes, then flip the turkey and cook for 5 minutes more.

Meanwhile, place the watercress and arugula in a salad bowl. Add the remaining raspberries, goat cheese, and walnuts halves into the bowl.

Use two folks to shred the turkey into small pieces and add to the salad bowl.

Pour over the dressing, then stir thoroughly to mix well.

Let the salad rest for 10 minutes, then serve.

STORAGE: Store in an airtight container in the fridge for 3 days.

REHEAT: Microwave, covered, until the turkey pieces are just warm.

SERVE IT WITH: To make this a delicious complete meal, serve it with keto burgers.

PER SERVING

calories: 553 | fat: 42.0g | total carbs: 12.1g | fiber: 4.9g | protein: 36.5g

Seared Rump Steak Salad

Macros: Fat 65% | Protein 27% | Carbs 8%

Prep time: 30 minutes | Cook time: 10 minutes | Serves 4

This hearty and satisfying rump steak salad is easy to prepare and is perfect for those warm summer evenings. It highly complements keto diet and goes well with keto bread to mop up the dressing and juices.

DRESSING:

- 2 teaspoons yellow mustard
- 1 tablespoon balsamic vinegar
- 2 tablespoons extra-virgin olive oil
- Salt and freshly ground black pvpper, to taste
- 8 ounces (227 g) rump steak
- 3 green onions, sliced
- 1 cup green beans, steamed and sliced
- 3 tomatoes, sliced
- 2 cups mixed salad greens
- 1 avocado, sliced

Make the dressing: Add yellow mustard, vinegar, oil, salt, and pepper in a medium mixing bowl. Mix until well combined. Set aside.

Preheat your grill pan to high heat.

Meanwhile, generously season the rump steak with salt and pepper in a separate bowl.

Sear the rump steak in the preheated pan for 4 minutes or until browned on each side.

Remove the steak from heat and let cool for 5 minutes. When cooled, thinly slice the steak.

Add green onions, green beans, tomatoes, and mixed salad greens to a salad bowl.

Pour the dressing into the salad bowl and toss until well mixed.

Top with avocado slices, then let rest for 5 minutes before serving.

STORAGE: Store in an airtight container in the fridge for 3 days.

REHEAT: Microwave the dressing and steak separately until just warm.

SERVE IT WITH: To make this a complete meal, you can serve it with grilled chicken thighs or pork chops.

PER SERVING

calories: 280 | fat: 20.2g | total carbs: 11.8g | fiber: 5.8g | protein: 18.6g

Sun-Dried Tomato and Feta Cheese Salad with Bacon

Macros: Fat 81% | Protein 15% | Carbs 4%

Prep time: 5 minutes | Cook time: 10 minutes | Serves 4

If you are looking for a fabulous salad to impress your guests or your family members, this sun-dried tomato and feta salad with bacon has got you covered. It is packed with nutrients and flavors.

- 5 ounces (142 g) bacon, chopped
- 5 sun-dried tomatoes in oil, sliced
- 1 cup feta cheese, crumbled
- 4 basil leaves
- 2 teaspoons extra-virgin olive oil
- 1 teaspoon balsamic vinegar Salt, to taste

Cook the bacon in a saucepan over medium heat for 4 minutes on each side, or until crisp and golden brown.

With a slotted spoon, transfer the bacon to a paper towel-lined plate to drain excess fat. Set aside.

Arrange the tomato slices in a salad bowl.

Scatter crumbled cheese and basil leaves over the tomatoes, then put the cooked bacon on top.

Drizzle the olive oil and vinegar over the mixture, then season with salt to taste.

Let the salad rest for 5 minutes to serve.

STORAGE: Store in an airtight container in the fridge for up to 3 days or in the freezer for up to 1 week.

REHEAT: Microwave the bacon, covered, until the desired temperature is reached or reheat the bacon in a frying pan or air fryer / instant pot, covered, on medium.

SERVE IT WITH: To make this a complete meal, you can serve it with grilled chicken thighs or pork chops.

PER SERVING

calories: 272 | fat: 24.7g | total carbs: 2.9g | fiber: 0.2g | protein: 10.0g

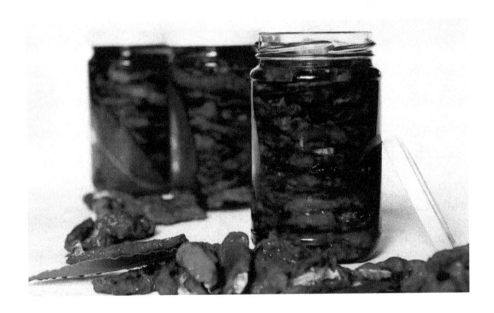

Chicken Salad with Parmesan Cheese

Macros: Fat 75% | Protein 19% | Carbs 6%

Prep time: 20 minutes | Cook time: 10 minutes | Serves 4

If you are looking forward to serving your family with a little different dinner meal, look no further. This chicken salad with Parmesan cheese is yummy, classic and the easiest chicken salad for hot summer days.

- 8 ounces (227 g) chicken thighs
- 2 garlic cloves, minced
- ¼ cup lemon juice
- 2 tablespoons olive oil
- 1head Romaine lettuce, torn
- 3 Parmesan cheese crisps
- ½ cup Parmesan cheese, grated

DRESSING:

- 2 tablespoons extra virgin olive oil
- 1 tablespoon lemon juice
- Salt and freshly ground black pepper, to taste

Place the chicken thighs, garlic, lemon juice, and olive oil in a sealable bag. Zip the bag and shake thoroughly until the chicken is well coated. Refrigerate the chicken for 1 hour to marinate.

Preheat your grill to medium-high heat.

Grill the marinated chicken for 4 minutes on each side. Remove from the grill and set aside.

Add the dressing ingredients in a mixing bowl and stir well to combine.

Arrange Romaine lettuce in a separate salad bowl and place cheese crisps on top. Pour the dressing over the lettuce and cheese crisps, then toss thoroughly until well coated.

Top the lettuce with the grilled chicken and grated cheese.

Let rest for 5 minutes and serve.

STORAGE: Store in an airtight container in the fridge for up to 2 days.

REHEAT: Microwave the chicken, covered, until the desired temperature is reached or reheat in a frying pan or air fryer / instant pot, covered, on medium.

SERVE IT WITH: To make this a complete meal, you can serve it with veggie skewers.

PER SERVING

calories: 328 | fat: 27.2g | total carbs: 8.8g | fiber: 3.4g | protein: 15.5g

Bacon, Smoked Salmon and Poached Egg Salad

Macros: Fat 81% | Protein 14% | Carbs 5%

Prep time: 10 minutes | Cook time: 15 minutes | Serves 4

Smoked salmon and poached egg make a stunning combination that can be served for lunch and a hearty filling breakfast.

DRESSING:

- 1 tablespoon lemon juice
- ½ cup mayonnaise, keto-friendly
- 1 teaspoon Tabasco sauce
- ½ teaspoon garlic purée
- 4 eggs
- 4 slices bacon
- 1 head Romaine lettuce, shredded
- ½ cup smoked salmon, sliced
- Salt and freshly ground black pepper, to taste

Add the dressing ingredients into a mixing bowl. Stir to combine well and set aside.

In a large saucepan, pour the water and sprinkle with a salt dash, then bring to a boil. One at a time, crack the eggs into the saucepan and cook for 3 minutes. Transfer the poached eggs to a plate and set aside.

 Cook the bacon slices in a skillet over medium heat for 8 minutes until crispy and well browned on both sides. Transfer to a separate plate lined with a paper towel, let drain and cool, and then chop into bite-sized pieces.

Add the lettuce, salmon, cooked bacon, and dressing to a large salad bowl. Sprinkle with salt and black pepper, then toss until well combined.

Divide the salad among 4 plates and top each plate with one poached egg.

Serve immediately or refrigerate to chill.

STORAGE: Store in an airtight container in the fridge for 2 days.

REHEAT: Microwave the bacon and salmon, if needed, covered, until the desired temperature is reached or reheat the bacon in a frying pan or air fryer

/ instant pot, covered, on medium.

SERVE IT WITH: To make this a complete meal, serve it with keto toast slices for a filling sandwich.

PER SERVING

calories: 489 | fat: 44.3g | total carbs: 6.9g | fiber: 3.3g | protein: 17.3g

Spinach Salad with Mustard Vinaigrette and Bacon

Macros: Fat 81% | Protein 8% | Carbs 11%

P rep time: 15 minutes | Cook time: 10 minutes | Serves 4

This is a delicious steakhouse-style spinach salad with a vinaigrette dressing that I have ever prepared. The salad looks complex but is very easy and quick to make.

- 2 bacon slices, chopped
- 1 cup spinach
- 1 spring onion, sliced
- ½ lettuce head, shredded
- 1 hard-boiled egg, chopped
- 1 avocado, sliced

VINAIGRETTE:

- ¼ teaspoon garlic powder
- 1 teaspoon Dijon mustard
- 1 tablespoon white wine vinegar
- 3 tablespoons olive oil
- Salt, to taste

Cook bacon in a nonstick skillet over medium heat for 8 minutes or until cooked and crispy. Remove from heat to plate lined with a paper towel to drain and cool. Set aside.

In a medium mixing bowl, add spinach, onion, lettuce, and chopped egg.

Stir to combine well.

Add all the vinaigrette ingredients in a separate bowl and whisk together until well mixed.

Pour the vinaigrette dressing over the spinach mixture and toss thoroughly until well coated.

Top with cooked bacon and avocado slices. Serve immediately.

STORAGE: Store in an airtight container in the fridge for 4 to 5 days.

REHEAT: Microwave the bacon, if needed, covered, until the desired temperature is reached or reheat the bacon in a frying pan or air fryer / instant pot, covered, on medium.

SERVE IT WITH: To make this a complete meal, serve it with sliced button mushrooms and fried chicken.

PER SERVING

calories: 273 | fat: 25.2g | total carbs: 8.2g | fiber: 4.8g | protein: 6.1g

Brussel Sprouts and Spinach Salad

Macros: Fat 77% | Protein 6% | Carbs 17%

P rep time: 10 minutes | Cook time: 25 minutes | Serves 4

Brussels sprouts, spinach, and hazelnuts combine to make a delicious salad that even the kids will enjoy eating. The combination of flavors and colors make this salad a perfect side dish for all summer.

- 1 pound (454 g) Brussels sprouts
- 4 tablespoons extra virgin olive oil, divided
- Salt and freshly ground black pepper, to taste
- ½ cup hazelnuts
- 1 cup baby spinach
- 1 tablespoon Dijon mustard
- 1tablespoon balsamic vinegar

Preheat your oven to 400°F (205°C). Line a baking pan with parchment paper and set aside.

Add Brussels sprouts in a mixing bowl, then drizzle with 2 tablespoons of olive oil and season with salt and pepper. Mix until the Brussels sprouts are well coated.

Spread the Brussels sprouts on the prepared baking pan and bake in the preheated oven for 20 minutes or until they are tender.

Meanwhile, toast hazelnuts in a heavy pan over medium heat for 2 minutes. Remove from heat and let cool, then chop into bite-sized pieces.

Once the Brussels sprouts are cooked, transfer them to a salad bowl. Add chopped hazelnuts, spinach, and Dijon mustard. Mix thoroughly until well combined.

In a separate bowl, add vinegar and remaining olive oil and mix thoroughly. Pour the mixture over the salad and gently toss to combine.

Let rest for 5 minutes and serve.

STORAGE: Store in an airtight container in the fridge for 5 days.

SERVE IT WITH: To make this a complete meal, serve it with grilled beef steak or chicken roast.

PER SERVING

calories: 258 | fat: 23.0g | total carbs: 11.7g | fiber: 4.7g | protein: 5.4g

Green Chicken Salad

Macros: Fat 71% | Protein 24% | Carbs 5%

Prep time: 10 minutes | Cook time: 15 minutes | Serves 4

This is a great way to cheer up your desire to chicken salad. The minty and chicken flavors takes the salad to the next level, making it perfect to please your crowd during a family gathering.

- 2 cups water
- 2 eggs
- 1 tablespoon avocado oil
- 1 chicken breast, cubed
- 2cups steamed green beans
- 4 cups mixed salad greens
- 1 avocado, sliced
- 2 tablespoons olive oil
- 2 tablespoons lemon juice
- 1 teaspoon Dijon mustard
- Salt and freshly ground black pepper, to taste
- 1 tablespoon mint, chopped

In a pot, add 2 cups of water, and sprinkle with a dash of salt, then stir to combine. Add the eggs into the pot and let boil over medium heat for 10 minutes.

Once the eggs are cooked, transfer to a bowl with cold water. Peel the eggs under the water and cut into medium-sized chunks.

Heat the avocado oil in a heavy skillet over medium heat and cook the chicken breast for 4 minutes. Remove from the heat and let cool, then slice.

Divide the steamed green beans and mixed salad greens between two salad bowls, then equally add the eggs, chicken, and avocado in both bowls.

In a separate bowl, add olive oil, lemon juice, and Dijon mustard, salt, and pepper, whisk until well mixed.

Drizzle the mustard mixture over the salad in the two salad bowls.

Top with chopped mint, then let rest for 5 minutes to serve.

STORAGE: Store in an airtight container in the fridge for up to 3 days.

REHEAT: Microwave the chicken, if needed, covered, until the desired temperature is reached or reheat in a frying pan or air fryer / instant pot, covered, on medium.

SERVE IT WITH: To make this a complete meal, serve it with tomato and egg drip soup or veggie skewers.

PER SERVING

calories: 373 | fat: 29.6g | total carbs: 10.1g | fiber: 5.9g | protein: 22.5g

Lettuce Wraps with Mackerel

Macros: Fat 44% | Protein 53% | Carbs 3%

Prep time: 10 minutes | Cook time: 20 minutes | Serves 4

It is quick and easy to make mackerel salad. Iit is also healthy and a great low- mercury alternative to tuna salad. The lettuce cups are perfect for light dinners and packed lunches.

- 2 mackerel fillets, sliced
- 1 tablespoon olive oil
- Salt and freshly ground black pepper, to taste
- 2 eggs
- 1tomato, deseeded and chopped
- 2 tablespoons keto-friendly mayonnaise
- ½ head lettuce, separated into leaves

Heat your heavy skillet over medium-high heat until hot.

Meanwhile, place the fish on a cutting board. Rub the fillets with olive oil, then season with salt and pepper.

Place the seasoned fish to the hot skillet and cook for 4 minutes on each side. Remove the fish from heat and set aside to cool.

In a pot, add 2 cups of salted water. Add the eggs and boil them for 10 minutes. Once cooked, remove the eggs from the pot to a bowl with cold water.

Peel the eggs and slice them into small pieces. Put the eggs in a salad bowl.

Add the fish, tomatoes, and mayo to the salad bowl. Use a spoon to mix thoroughly until well combined.

Layer a lettuce leaf as a cup on a platter and fill with 2 tablespoons of fish salad. Repeat the process with remaining lettuce leaves and fish salad.

Serve immediately.

STORAGE: Store in an airtight container in the fridge for 2 days.

SERVE IT WITH: To make this a complete meal, serve it with grilled beef steak or chicken roast.

PER SERVING

calories: 368 | fat: 18.1g | total carbs: 3.6g | fiber: 1.2g | protein: 45.5g

Iceberg Lettuce Salad with Bacon and Gorgonzola Cheese

Macros: Fat 78% | Protein 16% | Carbs 6%

Prep time: 9 minutes | Cook time: 6 minutes | Serves 4

The crunch lettuce leaves with the crisp bacon and cheese make this a sensational salad that will leave your taste buds delighted and asking for more.

- 4 ounces (113 g) bacon
- 1 tablespoon white wine vinegar
- 3 tablespoons extra virgin olive oil
- Salt and freshly ground black pepper, to taste
- 1 head iceberg lettuce, separated into leaves
- 1½ cups Gorgonzola cheese, crumbled
- 2 tablespoons pumpkin seeds

Place the bacon on a cutting board and chop it into bite-sized pieces.

Transfer the bacon to a nonstick skillet and cook over medium heat for 6 minutes or until the bacon is crispy and evenly browned.

Remove from heat and transfer to plate lined with paper towels to drain the excess fat and cool

Add vinegar, oil, salt, and pepper to a medium-sized mixing bowl. Using a spoon to stir thoroughly until the mixture is perfectly combined. Set aside.

Lay the lettuce leaves on a platter and top it with cooked bacon and cheese. Drizzle the vinegar mixture over the salad and toss until well coated.

Top the salad with pumpkin seeds, then let rest for 10 minutes to serve.

STORAGE: Store in an airtight container in the fridge for 2 days.

REHEAT: Microwave the bacon, if needed, covered, until the desired temperature is reached or reheat the bacon in a frying pan or air fryer / instant pot, covered, on medium.

SERVE IT WITH: To make this a complete meal, serve it with green and egg drip soup or veggie skewers.

PER SERVING

calories: 432 | fat: 37.9g | total carbs: 7.6g | fiber: 2.5g | protein: 17.2g

Beef, Pork, and Vegetable Salad with Yoghurt Dressing

Macros: Fat 63% | Protein 31% | Carbs 6%

Prep time: 15 minutes | Cook time: 15 minutes | Serves 4

A salad that is packed with vegetables and protein is all you need to energize the body. The beef, crisp vegetables with a yogurt dressing, is just perfect for a warm summer evening.

- 1 pound (454 g) ground beef
- 1 tablespoon fresh parsley, chopped
- 1 onion, grated
- 1whisked egg
- ½ teaspoon dried oregano
- ¼ cup pork rinds, crushed
- 1 garlic clove, minced
- Salt and freshly ground black pepper, to taste
- 2tablespoons olive oil, divided
- 1 cup arugula
- 1 cucumber, sliced
- 1 cup cherry tomatoes, halved
- 1½ tablespoons lemon juice
- 1 cup plain Greek yogurt
- 1 tablespoon fresh mint, chopped
- 2 tablespoons unsweetened almond milk

Add beef, parsley, onion, egg, oregano, pork rinds, garlic, salt, and pepper in a medium mixing bowl. Stir thoroughly until well mixed.

Use your hands to mold small balls with the mixture and place them on a clean work surface.

Heat half of the olive oil in a skillet over medium heat and cook the meatballs for 10 minutes on both sides or until well cooked. Remove the balls from heat and set aside on a plate lined with paper towels.

Add arugula, cucumber, and tomatoes in a salad bowl and mix well to combine. Stir in the remaining olive oil, lemon juice, salt, and pepper in the salad until well mixed.

In a separate bowl, whisk together Greek yogurt, mint, and almond milk until well mixed.

Pour the yogurt mixture over the salad and top with the meatballs. Serve immediately.

STORAGE: Store in an airtight container in the fridge for 3 days or freeze or up to a week.

REHEAT: Microwave the meat ball, if needed, covered, until the desired temperature is reached or reheat in a frying pan or air fryer / instant pot, covered, on medium.

SERVE IT WITH: To make this a complete meal, serve it with green soup, and pork and broccoli skewers.

PER SERVING

calories: 462 | fat: 32.3g | total carbs: 8.1g | fiber: 1.1g | protein: 35.9g

Crabmeat and Celery Salad

Macros: Fat 86% | Protein 11% | Carbs 3%

Prep time: 2 hours | Cook time: 0 minutes | Serves 6

It is a healthy seafood salad delicacy. You can have the salad alone or with company. It has an amazing fusion of flavors. And the fragrance of the celery will also give you a freshness eating enjoyment.

- ½ cup green bell pepper, diced
- ½ cup red onion, diced
- 1pound (454 g) flaked crab meat
- ½ cup celery, diced

DRESSING:

- 1½ cups keto-friendly mayonnaise
- ¼ cup sour cream
- 2tablespoons lemon juice
- ⅔ cup Italian salad dressing
- ½ teaspoon oregano, dried
- Salt and freshly ground black pepper, to taste

In a large bowl, add the diced green peppers, onions, crab meat, and celery and mix well. Set aside.

Make the dressing: In a separate bowl, add mayonnaise, sour cream, lemon juice, salad dressing, oregano, pepper and salt.

Pour the dressing into the bowl of crab mixture and gently toss to mix.

Cover the bowl with plastic wrap and let sit for 2 hours in the fridge.

Divide the salad among six plates and serve.

STORAGE: Store in an airtight container in the refrigerator for up to no more than 5 days.

SERVE IT WITH: To make this a complete meal, serve with creamy chicken.

PER SERVING

calories: 546 | fat: 53.2g | total carbs: 4.5g | fiber: 0.5g | protein: 14.3g

Cheesy Crab Stuffed Mushrooms

Macros: Fat: 75% | Protein: 21% | Carbs: 4%

Prep time: 15 minutes | Cook time: 17 minutes | Serves 6

A party favorite appetizer of stuffed mushrooms with a flavorsome filling... These mushrooms are stuffed with a flavorsome combination of crab meat, cream cheese, parmesan, almonds and herbs.

- 12 large button mushrooms, cleaned and stemmed
- 1 cup cooked crab meat, chopped
- 1 cup cream cheese, softened
- ½ cup Parmesan cheese, grated
- ¼ cup ground almonds
- 1 scallion, chopped
- 1 tablespoon fresh parsley, chopped
- 1 teaspoon garlic, minced
- Olive oil spray

Preheat the oven to 375°F (190°C) and line a baking sheet with parchment paper.

Arrange the mushrooms onto the prepared baking sheet, stem-side up. Lightly spray them with olive oil spray. Bake in the preheated oven for about 2 minutes. Remove from the oven to a plate lined with paper towels to drain the grease.

Meanwhile, make the filling: In a large bowl, place the remaining ingredients and mix until well combined. Stuff each mushroom with about 1½ tablespoons of the filling mixture. Arrange the stuffed mushrooms onto the same baking sheet.

Bake for about 14 to 15 minutes or until the mushrooms become bubbly and golden brown.

Remove the baking sheet from oven and serve warm.

STORAGE: You can store the filling in a container in the refrigerator for 1 to 2 days.

REHEAT: Microwave, covered, until the desired temperature is reached or reheat in a frying pan or air fryer / instant pot, covered, on medium.

SERVE IT WITH: Serve the stuffed mushrooms with the mashed broccoli or cauliflower.

PER SERVING

calories: 198 | fat: 15.9g | total carbs: 4.6g | fiber: 0.6g | protein: 10.2g

Sweet and Zesty Chicken Wings

Macros: Fat: 49% | Protein: 45% | Carbs: 6%

Prep time: 15 minutes | Cook time: 40 minutes | Serves 4

A lip-smacking recipe of sticky wings is ideal for a snack party! These chicken wings are baked in the oven until crispy and then coated with a sweet and zesty sauce.

WINGS:

- 2   pounds (907 g) chicken wings
- 2 tablespoons coconut oil, melted

SAUCES:

- 4 tablespoons butter
- 2 teaspoons garlic, minced
- 2 teaspoons fresh ginger, grated
- 2 to 3 tablespoons granulated monk fruit sweetener
- 3 to 4 tablespoons fresh lime juice
- 2 to 3 teaspoons lime zest, grated

Preheat the oven to 400°F (205°C) and line a baking sheet with parchment paper.

For the wings: In a large bowl, place the wings and coconut oil. Toss to coat well. Arrange the wings onto the prepared baking sheet in a single layer. Bake for about 40 minutes, flipping once halfway through.

Meanwhile, make the sauce: In a small saucepan, melt the butter over medium-high heat and sauté the garlic and ginger for about 3 minutes. Stir in the monk fruit sweetener, lime juice and zest, then bring to a gentle boil. Reduce the heat to medium and cook for about 10 to 15 minutes or until it reaches the desired thickness, stirring frequently. Remove the saucepan from heat.

Remove the wings from the oven to a large bowl. Pour the sauce over the wings and serve warm.

STORAGE: In a resealable plastic bag, place the baked and then cooled chicken wings. Seal the bag and refrigerate for about 3 to 4 days.

REHEAT: Microwave, covered, until the desired temperature is reached or reheat in a frying pan or air fryer / instant pot, covered, on medium.

PER SERVING

calories: 474 | fat: 26.4g | total carbs: 6.9g | protein: 50.1g | fiber: 0.1g

Hearty Bacon and Mushroom Platter

Macros: Fat: 49% | Protein: 19% | Carbs: 33%

Prep time: 15minutes | Cook time: 15 minutes | Serves 4

A one-pan family favorite recipe of bacon and mushrooms... This easy to cook but richly delicious dish is prepared with only 5 ingredients.

- 6 uncured bacon strips, chopped
- 4 cups fresh wild mushrooms, sliced
- 2 teaspoons garlic, minced
- 2 tablespoons homemade chicken stock
- 1 tablespoon fresh thyme, chopped

Heat a large nonstick skillet over medium-high heat and cook the bacon for about 7 minutes or until crispy, stirring frequently. Add the mushrooms and garlic and sauté for about 7 minutes. Add the chicken stock and with the wooden spoon, stir to scrape up any browned bits from the bottom of skillet.

Remove from the heat and serve hot with fresh thyme sprinkled on top.

STORAGE: Store in an airtight container in the fridge for up to 4 days or in the freezer for up to 1 month.

REHEAT: Microwave, covered, until the desired temperature is reached or reheat in a frying pan or air fryer / instant pot, covered, on medium.

SERVE IT WITH: Serve this dish with your favorite greens.

TIP: Topping of Parmesan cheese will enhance the flavor of bacon and mushrooms.

PER SERVING

calories: 67 | fat: 3.9g | total carbs: 6.0g | fiber: 2.6g | protein: 3.9g

Keto Smoked Salmon Fat Bombs

Macros: Fat 90% | Protein 10% | Carbs 0%

Prep time: 10 minutes | Cook time: 0 minutes | Serves 12 Fat Bombs

Salmon fat bombs are a combination of healthy fat like grass-fed butter, coconut oil, nut and the protein salmon. It provides an excellent keto diet with the low-carb content.

- ½ cup goat cheese, at room temperature
- 2 teaspoons freshly squeezed lemon juice
- 2 ounces (57 g) smoked salmon
- Freshly ground black pepper, to taste
- ½ cup butter, at room temperature

Line a baking sheet with parchment paper and set aside.

Make the fat bombs: In a bowl, add cheese, lemon juice, smoked salmon, pepper, and butter, then stir well to blend.

Scoop 1 tablespoon of the butter mixture onto the baking sheet until you make 12 equally sized mounds.

Transfer the sheet into the refrigerator for about 3 hours until fat bombs become firm.

Remove from the refrigerator and let stand under room temperature for a few minutes before serving.

STORAGE: Store in an airtight container in the fridge for up to 4 days or in the freezer for up to 1 month.

SERVE IT WITH: To make this a complete meal, you can serve it with plain Greek yogurt.

PER SERVING

calories: 88 | fat: 9.0g | total carbs: 0g | fiber: 0g | protein: 1.9g

Deviled Eggs with Bacon And Cheese

Macros: Fat 80% | Protein 16% | Carbs 4%

Prep time: 15 minutes | Cook time: 0 minutes | Serves 12

The deviled eggs contain finely shredded Swiss cheese and bacon. They are nutritionally better than ordinary eggs. The recipe is easy and takes a short duration of time to cook.

- 6 large hard-boiled eggs, peeled
- ¼ cup keto-friendly mayonnaise
- ¼ cup finely shredded Swiss cheese
- ½ teaspoon Dijon mustard
- ¼ chopped avocado
- Ground black pepper, to taste
- 6 cooked and chopped bacon slices

Cut the eggs in halves. Spoon the yolk out carefully and put in a bowl.

Arrange the whites, hollow side facing up, on a plate.

Crumble the yolks with a fork. Add the mayonnaise, cheese, mustard, and avocado. Stir well to mix. Add the pepper to season.

Fill the hollow egg whites with the yolk mixture.

Top every egg half with the bacon before serving.

STORAGE: Store in an airtight container in the fridge for up to 4 days or in the freezer for up to 1 month.

REHEAT: Microwave, covered, until it reaches the desired temperature.

SERVE IT WITH: To make this a complete meal, serve with broccoli Cheddar soup.

PER SERVING

calories: 134 | fat: 11.9g | total carbs: 1.45g | fiber: 0.3g | protein: 5.2g

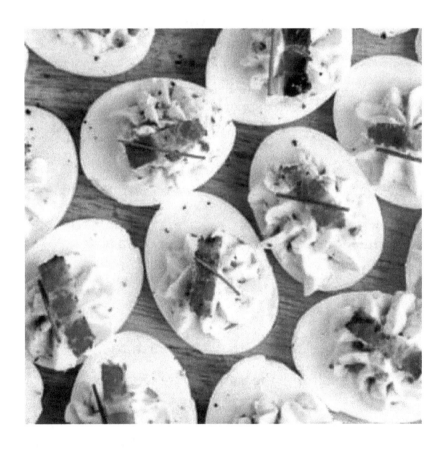